Love Notes
TO MY SISTAS

A journal and workbook designed for healing, wellness and love. I want your soul to prosper and soar.

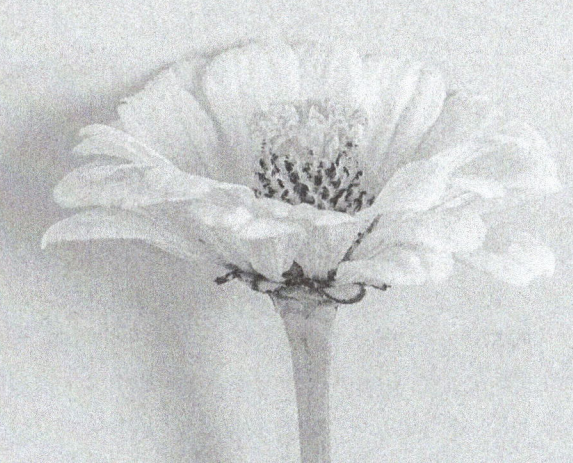

SHAAREE M. MCCALPINE

MEET YOUR COACH

I started writing this journal/workbook to help you cope with life's struggles. Along the way, it helped me with hurts and the struggle to be who I am and still have relationships I thought I valued in my life. See, I've always been a dope chick, people always wanted to be around me and draw from my energy and dopeness. Problem was, once they were in the gravitational pull they couldn't handle it. They began to want to dull my shine, pull me down and lessen my God given ability to be a force and a voice.

Lol, go figure the things that "people" would complain about, like she is too loud, turn it down, you talk too much, you too sarcastic now brings me a hefty wage, and some of the same people ask for advice or need my services. Any who, where was I? Oh yeah, sis I'm here to change the definition of strong black women. It's not the image of struggle, anxious and depressed.

For me, I want the strong black women to be a narrative of courage, moving in a way that supports your God given gifts. Not minimizing to make others, by others anybody that tries to silence you or make you feel less than, feel comfortable. I love you and hope that my words and deeds can help you. Being strong sis means I think I can and trying regardless of the fear or your naysayers. If you don't get it right the first time, it's cool, as long as you are breathing you get a chance to try again. That right there is strength, Trust that my baby.

We as black women, tend to look to friends and family for support, listen sometimes they can't imagine or don't want you to succeed nevertheless it's not their job. Move as if the entire world supports you because it does, our Devine creator is waiting for you to Boss up. TD Jakes said something that sticks with me to this day "I never met a hater that was doing better than me". Facts people on your level or above got other ish to do. Sis, I know it's hard out there but that doesn't mean it can't be done. The adventure starts today. Don't be afraid to knock all this shit over, lesss go!

Shaaree xoxo

Workbook
Inside

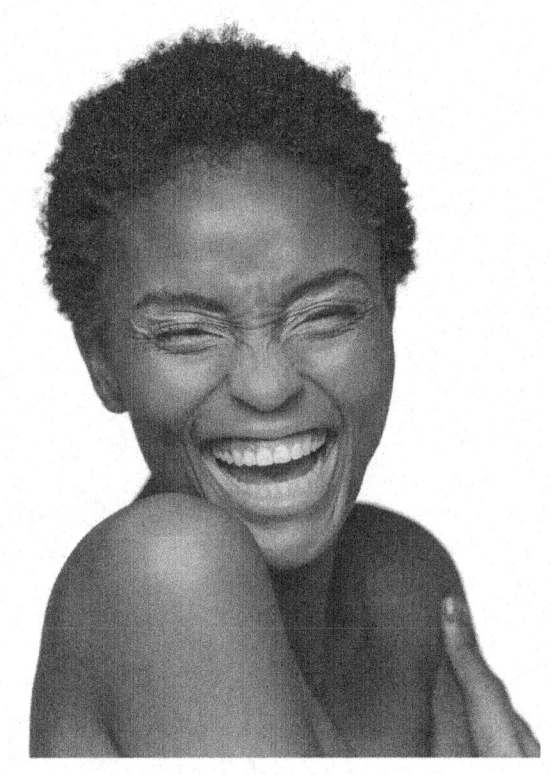

Faith Soars workbook will provide you with a practical step-by-step guide on how to soar and become a better YOU!

01 STRESS

Stress is a feeling of emotional or physical tension. Too much stress can be debilitating. You will learn specific techniques for managing stress more effectively so that you can enjoy life.

02 ANXIETY

Anxiety is a feeling of fear, dread, and uneasiness. Anxiety can cause you to feel restless, stressed, and a rapid heart rate, etc. You will learn how to manage anxiety and live fearlessly!

03 DEPRESSION

Depression is a mood disorder that causes a persistent feeling of sadness and loss of interest. You will learn how limiting beliefs will determine what you think is possible and how you react to obstacles.

04 GRIEF & LOSS

Grief is a natural response to loss. There are five stages of grief and loss. You will learn that pain eases over time and that it is possible to accept loss and move forward in life.

05 HEALTHY RELATIONSHIPS

Healthy relationships are made up of respect, honesty, trust, and communication. You will learn how to break the cycle of unhealthy relationships and learn how to form healthy relationships moving forward.

You don't have
to be great
to start
But you have
to start to be
great.

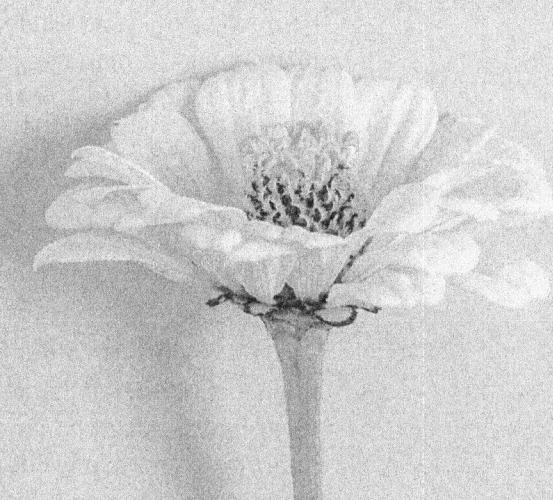

01 STRESS

Stress is a feeling of being strained, overwhelmed, and exhausted. A minimal amount of stress is considered motivating, however, if too much stress occurs it can make less strenuous tasks such as taking out the trash seem overwhelming. If small tasks accumulate over time, it can lead to a massive blow up that can result in major problems.

Stressors include daily nuisances, life changes or life circumstances. Things that can protect you against stress includes positive coping strategies, daily mood boosters, and protective contributions like implementing healthy boundaries.

peace be still

STRESS INSPECTION

This activity will help you understand how your daily habits contribute to your biggest challenges. Describe your biggest pain points in each of the following categories and rate them on a scale of 1-4, where 1 is "extremely stressful" and 4 is "a little stressful". Are you surprised by the stressors that contribute to your larger challenges?

Daily Mood Stressors
Common strains that negatively impacts daily life.
Examples: *work problems, lack of sleep, limited free time, argument with partner*

1.
2.
3.
4.

Major Life Changes
Important events that require significant adjustment in your life.
Examples: *separation or divorce, new job, moving, grief and loss*

1.
2.
3.
4.

Life Circumstances
Long-term circumstances that contributes to life being more difficult.
Examples: *financial problems, chronic illness, toxic relationships, job dissatisfaction*

1.
2.
3.
4.

Part Two
STRESS INSPECTION

In the last activity, you identified your biggest pain points. Now, think about how you can incorporate healthy coping mechanisms for each of your pain points into your daily routine. **Keeping a daily routine helps you to stay organized and focused, it also helps you achieve work-life harmony.** Consider the factors that protect you against stress, such as getting your rest, exercising, eating a healthy meal or speaking with a professional about your problems.

Daily Mood Boosters
Positive people, places or things that creates joy and happiness.
Examples: daily affirmations, surrounding yourself with loving people, eating a good meal

1.
2.
3.
4.

Healthy Coping Mechanisms
Important activities that reduces stress in your life and embraces happiness.
Examples: exercise, yoga, swimming, dance, journaling

1.
2.
3.
4.

Positive Contributions
Life circumstances that protect you from stress.
Examples: good health, supportive family and friends, motivation to succeed, therapist

1.
2.
3.
4.

Weekly Success Planner

In the first activity, you identified your pain points, then you made a list of healthy coping mechanisms to protect you from stress. Weekly planning prevents you from experiencing additional stress from factors that are outside of your control. In this example, you will learn how to create a long-term goal, identify the weekly priorities to help you reach the goal, and identify why the priorities are important to you.

Sis, let's plan for success!

Long Term Goal/s: usually take 12 months or more to achieve

make your weekly priorities align with this goal:

complete my college degree

My weekly priorities:

01 Plan homework/study times for every course

02 Meet with English professor to review last research paper

03 Update weekly planner with deadlines for important exams and homework assignments

Why they're important to me:

Scheduling study time will help me achieve good grades

I will learn the mistakes I made during my last term paper and improve my writing skills

Staying on top of important deadlines on my homework assignments and exams will help me be prepared

Potential Distractions

Getting sidetracked by social media

How to Avoid Them

Silence notifications on my phone while studying or doing homework

Other Notes

Remember to reward yourself for a successful week!

Weekly Success Planner

Weekly planning will keep you motivated, help you perform at a higher level, measuring your progress, and most of all it will help you prioritize. Use this blank template to identify a long-term goal, your weekly priorities and why they're important to you. Once you have completed the activity, consider purchasing a yearly calendar to help you practice effective time management. Sis, let's plan for success!

Long Term Goal/s: usually take 12 months or more to achieve

make your weekly priorities align with this goal:

My Weekly Priorities:

01.

02.

03.

Why they're Important to me:

Potential Distractions

How to Avoid Them

Other Notes

" HEBREWS 6

17 Wherein God, willing more abundantly to shew unto the heirs of promise the immutability of his counsel, confirmed it by an oath:

18 that by two immutable things, in which it was impossible for God to lie, we might have a strong consolation, who have fled for refuge to lay hold upon the hope set before us:

19 which *hope* we have as an anchor of the soul, both sure and stedfast, and which entereth into that within the veil;

20 whither the forerunner is for us entered, even Jesus, made an high priest for ever after the order of Melchisedec.

be hopeful

Habit Tracker
31-day

This tool is a visual aid that reminds you to work towards your goals. As you see the progress you're making towards your goals, it will motivate you to achieve more. Most of all, using a habit tracker will give you a sense of satisfaction as you see a record of your success. Below you will see an example of pre-populated habits that you can try-out over the next 31-days. A brown circle indicates the habit has been completed.

	Reading	Yoga	Cooking	Work Out	Walking	Meditate	Mindfulness	Journal	Therapy	Family Time
01	●		●		●		●			
02										
03			●							
04	●									
05			●		●			●		
06										
07	●		●							
08										
09										
10	●									
11										
12										
13										
14										
15										
16										
17										
18										
19										
20										
21										
22										
23										
24										
25										
26										
27										
28										
29										
30										
31										

Your Turn!
Habit Tracker

Now it's your turn. In the last activity, you learned that this tool is a visual aid that reminds you to act. As you see the progress you're making towards your goals, it will motivate you to achieve more. Most of all, using a habit tracker will give you a sense of satisfaction as you see a record of your success. Over the next 31-days, add a habit you would like to try in the black fields. Once you complete the habit, populate the designated cell with a circle or 'x' to indicate that it is complete. You can add a total of 10 habits. You got this!

01										
02										
03										
04										
05										
06										
07										
08										
09										
10										
11										
12										
13										
14										
15										
16										
17										
18										
19										
20										
21										
22										
23										
24										
25										
26										
27										
28										
29										
30										
31										

Session Reflection

During this session, you learned about your biggest pain points, identified healthy coping mechanisms to combat challenges, and learned how to incorporate successful habits into your daily routine. Now, it is time to reflect on what you have learned and how you can implement healthy activities into your daily routine for a successful future. Below, ask yourself these questions and use the designated area to share your thoughts.

- What do I want the next few months look and feel like?
- What tools and resources do I need to make the next few months amazing?
- Based on my answers, what is going to be my top 3 priorities for the next 3-6 months?

02 ANXIETY

Anxiety is a mental and physical reaction to feelings of fear or uneasiness. In small doses, it can protect us from danger, and focuses our attention on problems. Anxiety can cause physical reactions in the body like sweat, feel tense or restless. Anxiety may drive people to avoid the things that scare them as well. It is the brain's way of reacting to stress and alerting you of potential danger.

Keep in mind that when a "scary" thing is avoided, there is an immediate sense of relief. However, the next time this feeling arises, it feels scarier. This creates a harmful cycle of avoidance and worsens anxiety. Symptoms of anxiety may include avoidance of fear, muscle tension, uncontrollable worry, upset stomach, sleep problems, or poor concentration.

prayer works

ANXIETY

Occasional anxiety is a normal part of life. Sometimes the feelings of anxiety can interfere with daily activities, can be difficult to control, and can last for longer periods of time. Use this activity to understand how you feel when your anxiety starts, and avoid places or situations to prevent these feelings.

HOW DO YOU FEEL WHEN YOU'RE MOST ANXIOUS?

- [ ] Slightly worried but functioning as usual
- [ ] Madly growing fear and stress
- [ ] Can't focus and overthinking
- [ ] Nearing anxiety attack
- [ ] Losing Control with physical discomfort

WHAT TYPICALLY HAPPENS THAT CAUSES MY ANXIETY?

_____

_____

WHAT FACTORS MAY INCREASE MY RISK OF ANXIETY?

Examples:
not meeting expectations at work, supporting family financially, not communicating my boundaries

FAITH SOARS

How this works

Mindfulness Reduces Anxiety

Research has shown that mindfulness helps reduce anxiety. Mindfulness teaches us how to respond to stress with self-awareness rather than simply acting with emotion. To get you where you're going, we must first understand what role anxiety plays in your life. Below is a simplified roadmap of a decision making process. You can either make all your important decisions on autopilot without actually being aware of them (on the left) or you can take a more mindful approach and take some time to reflect before reacting. Think about how you react to events, do you make deceision on autopilot or do you take a more mindful approach?

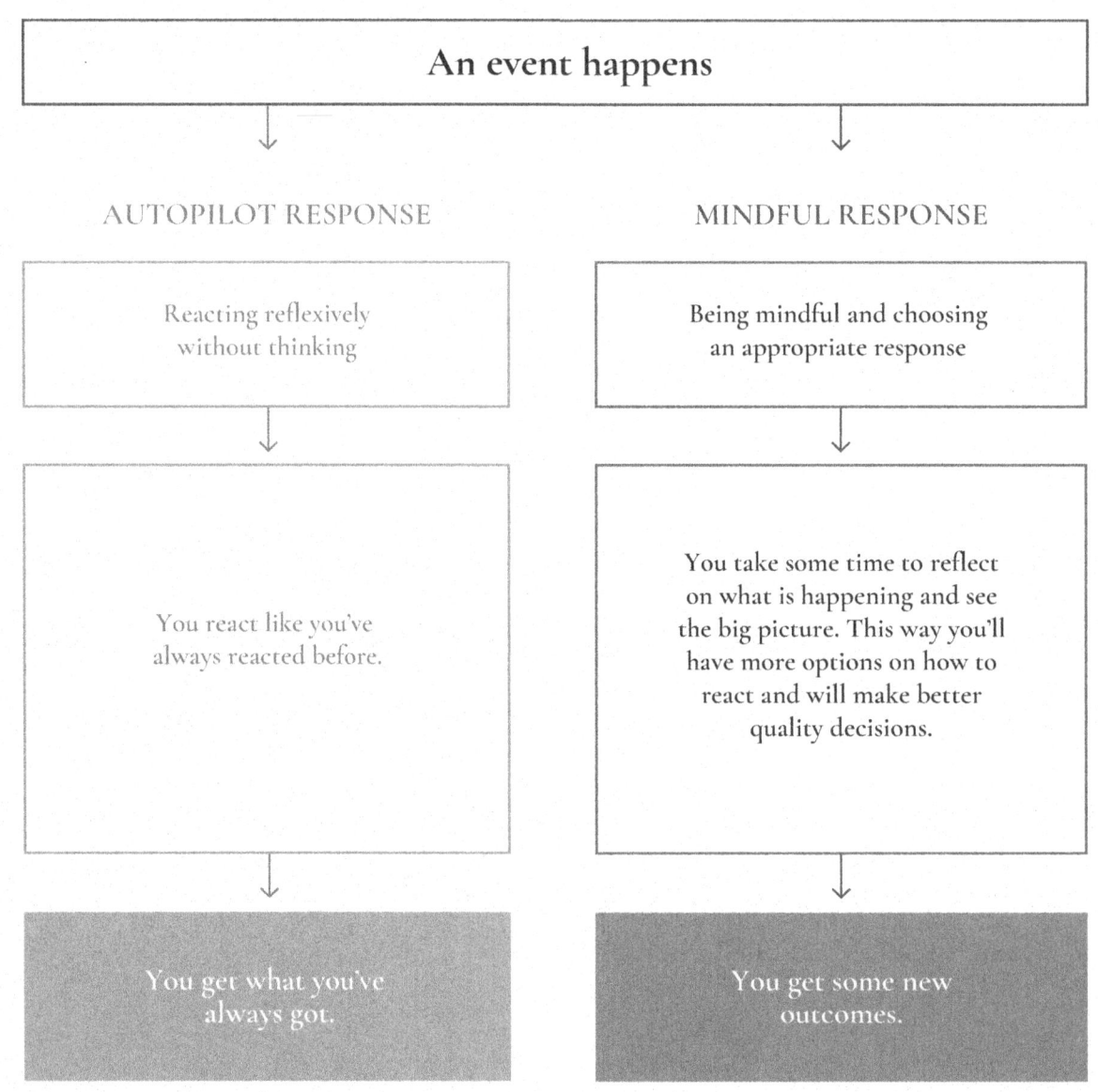

WWW.FAITHSOARSCOUNSELING.COM

Your turn!
Mindfulness Activity

Making intentional decisions can reduce anxiety. Use this simplified roadmap of a decision making process to identify how you can become more aware of your thoughts before reacting. This will help you identify some habitual patterns (typical reactions to situations) that most of the time get you the same results and trigger anxiety. On the other hand, by being mindful, you'll be able to make different decisions that will ultimately yield different outcomes and help you stay in the present moment.

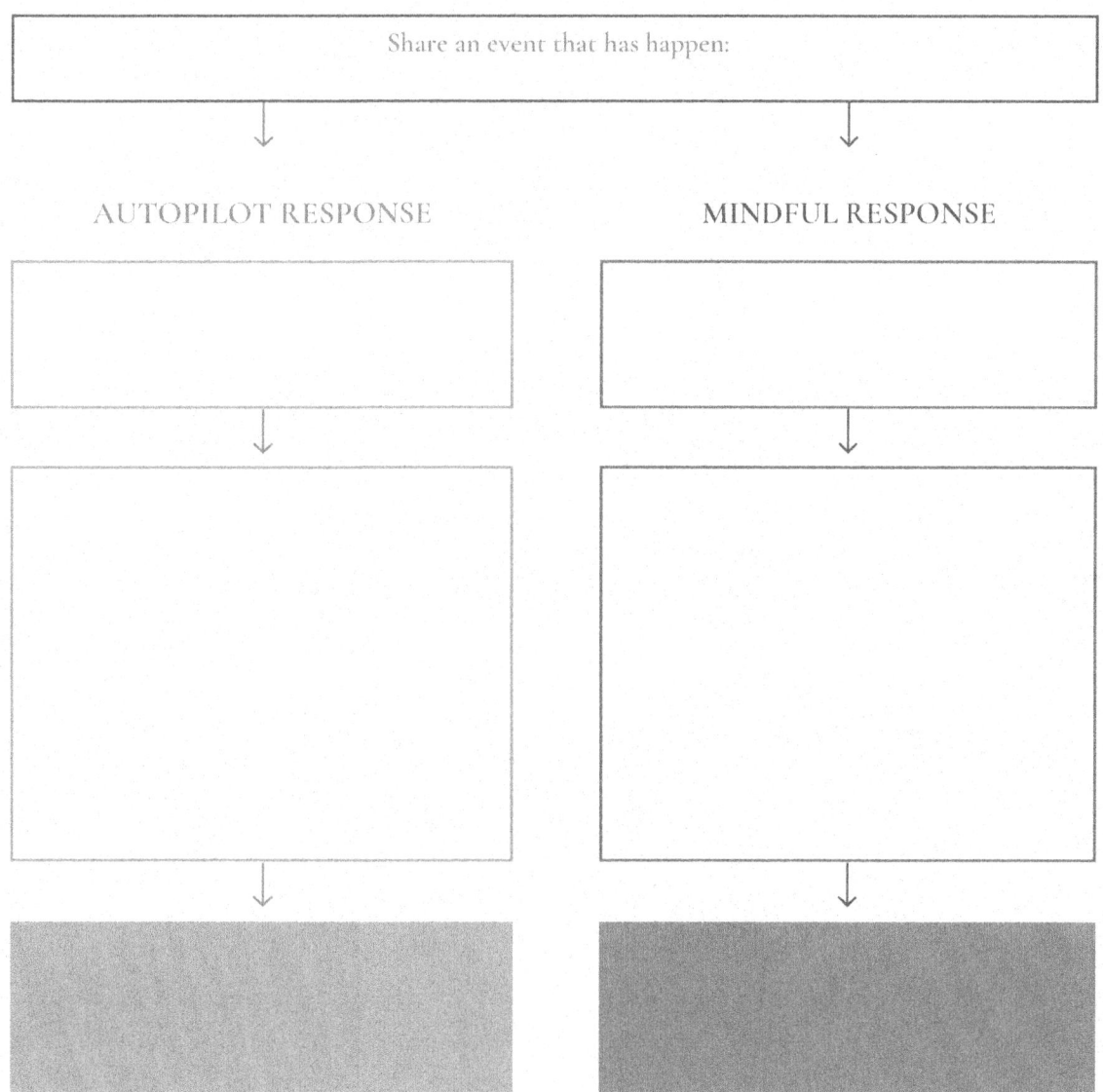

DAILY Mindfulness

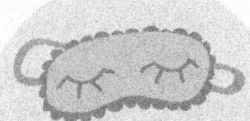
GET A GOOD SLEEP

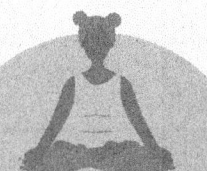
5 MINUTE MEDITATION

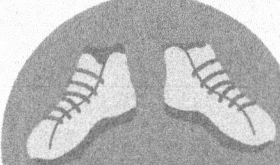
GO FOR A WALK

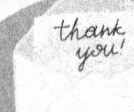
SAY THANK YOU

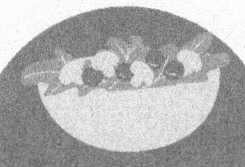
EAT MINDFULLY

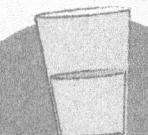
DRINK ENOUGH WATER

" PHILIPPIAN

4 Rejoice in the Lord alway: *and* again I say, Rejoice.

5 Let your moderation be known unto all men. The Lord is at hand.

6 Be careful for nothing; but in every thing by prayer and supplication with thanksgiving let your requests be made known unto God.

7 And the peace of God, which passeth all understanding, shall keep your hearts and minds through Christ Jesus.

peace of of God

Weekly Success Planner

Weekly planning will keep you motivated, help you perform at a higher level, measuring your progress, and most of all it will help you prioritize. Use this blank template to identify a long-term goal, your weekly priorities and why they're important to you. Once you have completed the activity, consider purchasing a yearly calendar to help you practice effective time management. Sis, let's plan for success!

Long Term Goal/s: usually take 12 months or more to achieve

make your weekly priorities align with this goal:

My Weekly Priorities: | **Why they're Important to me:**

01

02

03

Potential Distractions | **How to Avoid Them**

Other Notes

Session Reflection

During this session, you learned about how your body reacts to feelings of fear or uneasiness known as anxiety. You learned that anxiety can interfere with your daily activities and you identified what factors trigger your anxiety. Most importantly, you learned how to incorporate positive coping mechanisms like mindfulness into your daily routine to reduce anxiety. Reflect on what you have learned and how you can enhance your life by incorporating mindfulness exercises. Below, ask yourself these questions and use the designated area to share your thoughts.

- What is an event that triggers my anxiety and how would I typically respond.
- How can I respond differently moving forward?
- What mindfulness technique can I incorporate to cope with this stressful situation?

WWW.FAITHSOARSCOUNSELING.COM

03 DEPRESSION

According to the National Institute of Mental Health, **depression** is a common but serious mood disorder. It causes severe symptoms that affect how you may feel, think, and handle daily activities, such as sleeping, eating, or working. There are four main types of depression, such as persistent depressive disorder, psychotic depression, seasonal depression, and bipolar disorder.

Women are **2x more likely** to experience depression. About 1 in 10 people will experience depression during a lifetime. There are a few risks for depression to keep in mind such as family history, unemployment, social isolation and substance abuse.

Possible treatments to consider for depression is Cognitive Behavioral Therapy (CBT) and medication. CBT helps by shifting self-defeating thoughts and behaviors. Medication helps increase or decrease levels of chemicals in the brain. A combination of both CBT and medication has been found to be the most effective treatment for depression. Consult a professional for help that is specifically tailored to your needs.

God is with you

SIGNS & SYMPTOMS OF DEPRESSION

According to the National Institute of Mental Health (NIMH), an estimated **19.4 million adults** in the U.S had at least one major depressive episode. Use this checklist to identify the signs and symptoms of depression occurring in your life.

FEELINGS

- [ ] Sad, mood, dependency, despair or low self-esteem
- [ ] Physical aches and pains such as headaches or stomachaches
- [ ] Hard time sleeping or too much sleep
- [ ] Extreme sensitivity to (*and easily upset about*) things that happen
- [ ] Irritability, anger, or hostility
- [ ] Difficulty concentrating

THOUGHTS

- [ ] Thoughts of not being worth anything, or not being lovable
- [ ] Hopeless that things can change
- [ ] Believe cannot change things for the better
- [ ] Not interested in socializing with friends
- [ ] Thinking it would be better to be dead, thoughts of killing yourself
- [ ] No interest in doing things you use to enjoy doing

BEHAVIOR

- [ ] Withdrawing, stopped doing much of anything
- [ ] Poor communication, crying about little things or crying a lot
- [ ] Talking about or trying to run away from home
- [ ] Alcohol or substance abuse
- [ ] Hurting yourself on purpose, suicide attempt
- [ ] Absences from school or a drop in school performance

Limiting Beliefs

If you've experienced depression and anxiety, it is likely that you have developed limited beliefs which can chip away at your sense of self as well as your ability to cope and recover. Your belief system will determine what you think is possible and how you react to obstacles, therefore identifying any limiting beliefs you currently hold and actively reframing them is a key component to your long term success. Think about your limiting beliefs and the results you get by thinking in that manner.

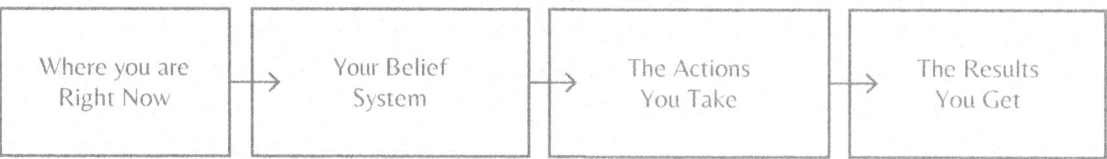

Where you are Right Now → Your Belief System → The Actions You Take → The Results You Get

What beliefs are currently holding me back?
Example: "I am not good enough to achieve what we want"

How are my beliefs different then those that my family and friends hold?
Example: "My family is pretty optimistic and I am realistic. They believe anything is possible for me, but I have children and real bills that have prevented me from achieving my goals"

How are these beliefs harmful? Are they even true?
Example: "These beliefs are harmful because it's stopping me from moving forward and growing on a personal and professional level"

What would you do if you would not be able to fail?
Example: "I would get my college degree and purchase my dream home"

What are some better and more productive alternatives for these beliefs?
- Life is good
- I'm confident
- People always like me
- I can do anything I want to do

WWW.FAITHSOARSCOUNSELING.COM

Your turn! Limiting Beliefs

In the last activity, you learned about the negative impact of limiting beliefs. Think about your limiting beliefs and the results you get by thinking in that manner. Now, it's your turn to share the beliefs that you feel are holding you back. How are those beliefs different from your family beliefs? How are they harmful? What would you do if you would not fail? Most of all, what are some better and productive alternatives for your beliefs?

| Where you are Right Now | → | Your Belief System | → | The Actions You Take | → | The Results You Get |

What beliefs are currently holding me back?

How are my beliefs different then those that my family and friends hold?

How are these beliefs harmful? Are they even true?

What would you do if you would not be able to fail?

What are some better and more productive alternatives for these beliefs?

WWW.FAITHSOARSCOUNSELING.COM

Breaking Negative Belief Cycles

At times, you may think negatively. You may have a bad day or feel like the world is against you. If you're not mindful, you may start to believe that things are intentionally harder for you or that others may not have the best intentions for you. The more you allow yourself to think negatively, the more negative thoughts you will have and it will become harder to break the negative cycle. Take a look this belief cycle below. Think about the role your negative experiences play in your negative belief cycle and answer the belief question below.

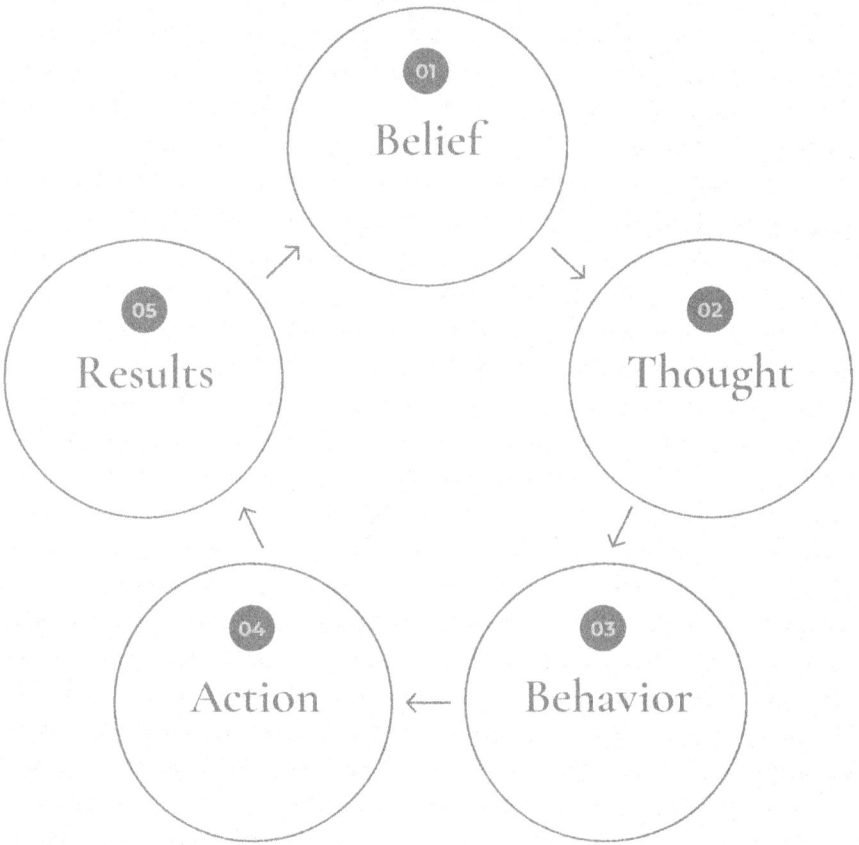

What steps will I take to break the negative belief cycle and start reenforcing positive beliefs, actions and results?

> **1 CORINTHIANS**

4 Love is patient, love is kind. It does not envy, it does not boast, it is not proud

5 It does not dishonor others, it is not self-seeking, it is not easily angered, it keeps no record of wrongs.

6 Love does not delight in evil but rejoices with the truth.

7 It always protects, always trusts, always hopes, always perseveres.

God loves me

Belief-Results Cycle

Although, there is no right answer to how to break a negative belief cycle, the first step is to identify the belief that is holding you back in the first place. The most effective way of breaking the cycle is either consciously altering your thoughts or being mindful of your actions - mostly because these two are directly in your control when you're being mindful enough and are thus the easiest to alter.

Also note that this cycle can also reenforce positive beliefs and actions once you break the negativity cycle. On this worksheet, you'll try to identify other beliefs that are holding you back and how you can reframe them to be more productive. For example, you may have thought when you were little that "Im not good enough". While it's true in a sense (because you hadn't reached your full potential), a more productive way of thinking would be that "I am worthy", "I am confident", "I am a good person that deserves good things".

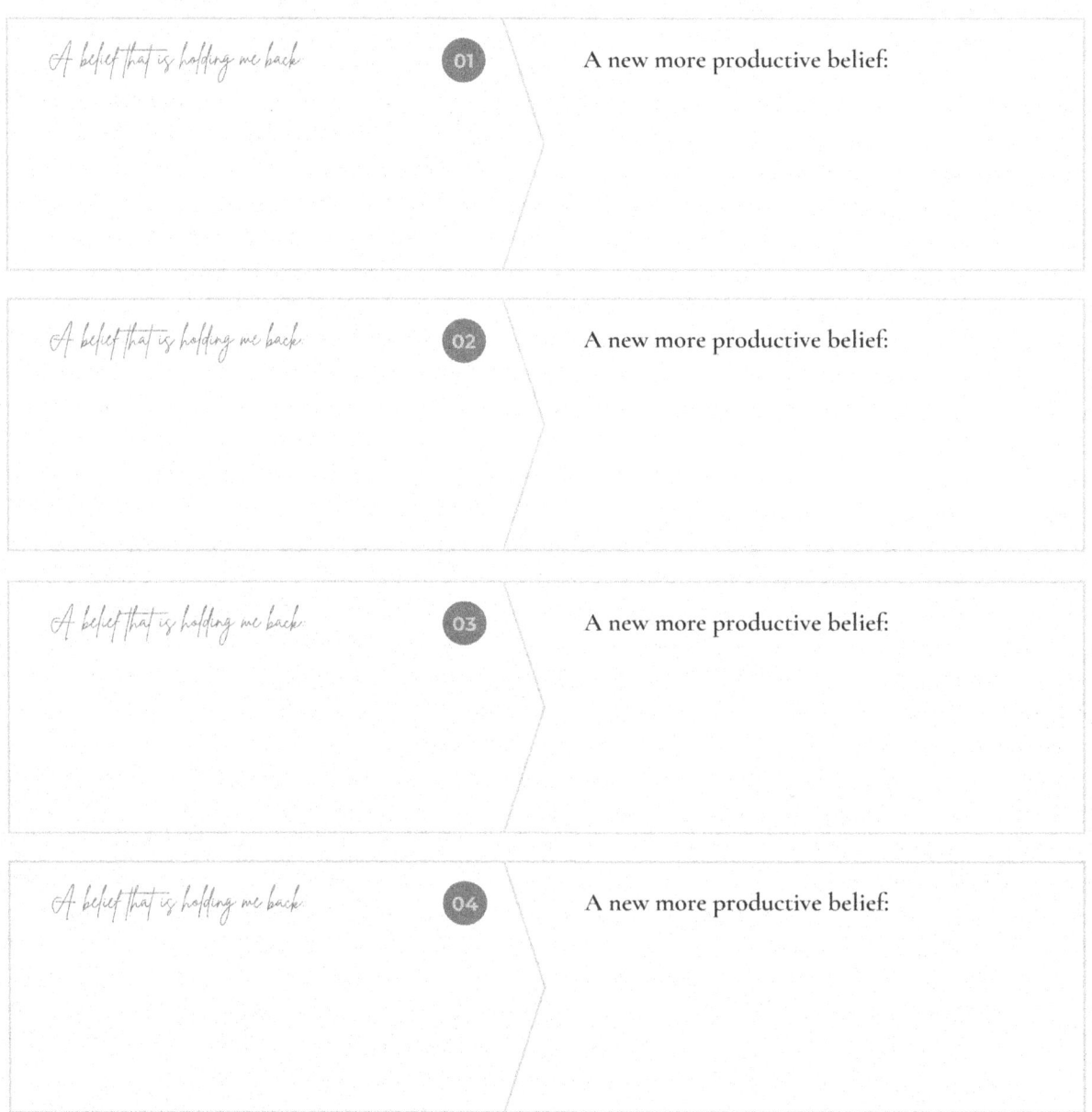

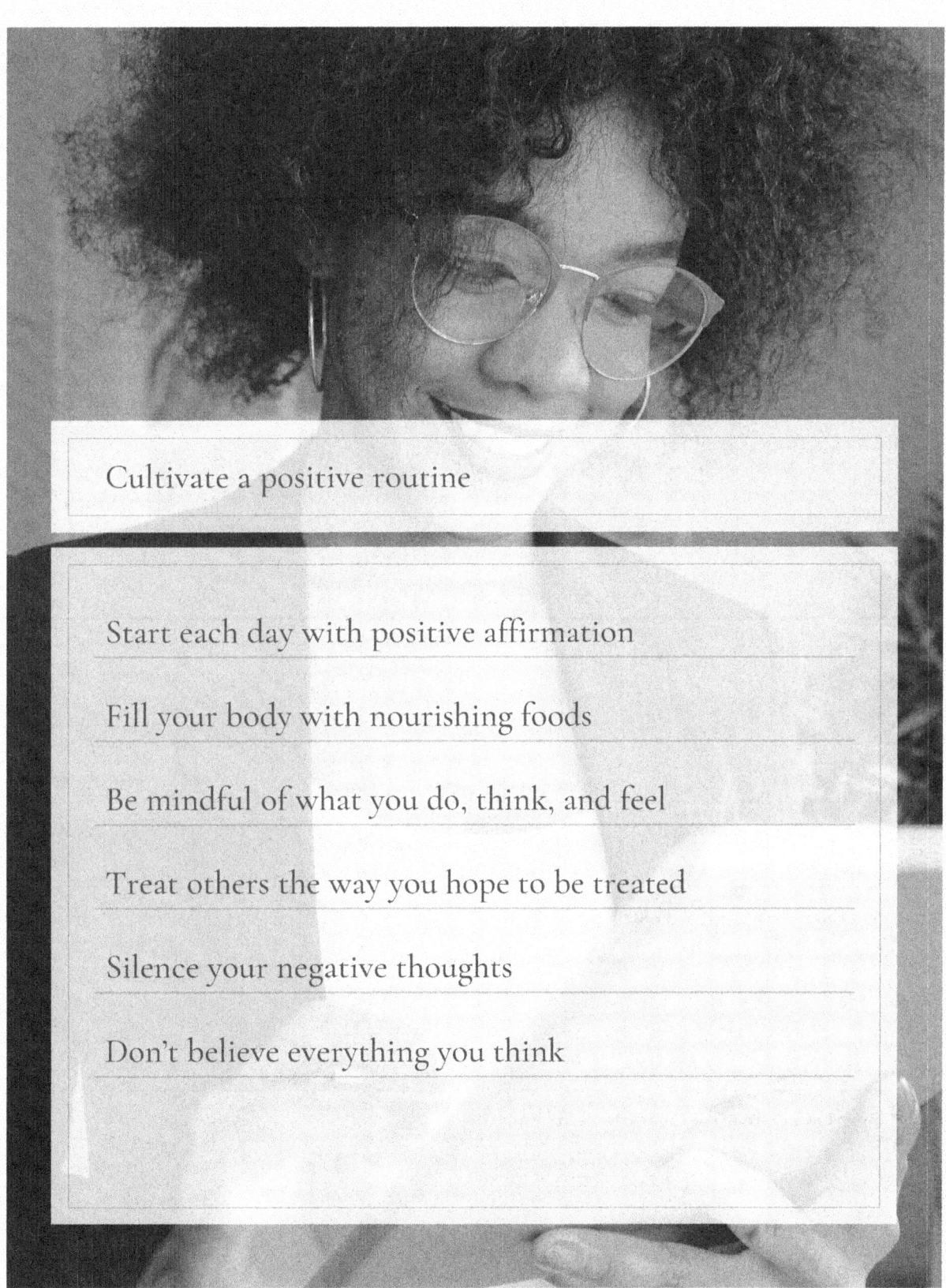

Cultivate a positive routine

- Start each day with positive affirmation
- Fill your body with nourishing foods
- Be mindful of what you do, think, and feel
- Treat others the way you hope to be treated
- Silence your negative thoughts
- Don't believe everything you think

Gratitude Journal

Morning:

I am greatful for:

I'm looking forward to:

Daily Affirmations:

Evening:

Good things that happened today:

Things I can do to make tomorrow even better:

WWW.FAITHSOARSCOUNSELING.COM

Session Reflection

During this session, you learned about that women are 2x more likely to experience depression as well as the signs and symptoms of depression. You learned that limiting beliefs can greatly impact your positive perspective of the world and how to break a negative belief cycle. Reflect on what you have learned and how you can enhance your life by incorporating a healthy belief cycle. Below, ask yourself these questions and use the designated area to share your thoughts.

- What are 5 positive core beliefs about myself? For example: "Life is good", "I'm healthy", "I'm confident"
- What are 3 practical ways that I can escape negative thinking such as, avoid all-or-nothing thinking or managing my expectations
- How can I incorporate positive core beliefs into my daily routine?

04
GRIEF & LOSS

Grief and Loss is the thoughts, feelings, and behaviors connected to the loss of something or someone important. The loss could be a death, a job, a relationship or anything a person values. Everyone deals with death differently. Some may cry for days, others may appear numb to their emotions. This portion of the workbook will help you identify how you grieve as well as helpful ways to mourn.

You will learn the grieving process, the five stages of grief as well as how to identify how you are currently navigating or will navigate your mourning process.

God is strength

GRIEF PROCESS

Grief is a natural process that can be painful, but personal and totally normal. During the grief process, you will learn about the different forms of grief and how it may impact your life. This process might trigger emotions that you are not familiar with and that is okay. Take a look at the grieving process below and give yourself permission to feel and heal.

ACUTE GRIEF

Immediately after a loss, it is normal to experience intense symptoms of shock, sadness, sleep issues, and poor concentration. Over time, these symptoms will diminish.

COMPLICATED GRIEF

The loss of a loved one can seem unimaginable for quite some time. This process can last for years and you might experience guilt about the idea of "moving on".

INTEGRATED GRIEF

At this point, you have accepted the reality of loss and resumed daily activities. This does not negate the fact that you miss your loved one, rather you aren't experiencing pain at their memory. You have learned how to cope, however, the likelihood of grief showing up during the holidays are very high.

NOTES

FIVE STAGES OF GRIEF & LOSS

Take a look at this five-step framework that makes up how we learn to live with the loss of a loved one. Think about how you felt when you first learned about the love one you lost. What stage are you currently in? Which start is the most difficult for you? What have you learned about yourself during this stage?

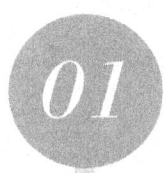

DENIAL

During the early stages of grief, some people might feel numb to their emotions. It is difficult to accept that a loved one is not coming back. It is common to feel the presence of someone who has passed as well.

ANGER

Natural emotions like anger is normal to experience during this stage in the grieving process. Death is unfair, especially when you had plans for the future with the loved one. It is common to feel angry towards the person who has died as well.

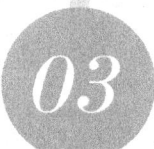

BARGAINING

It is difficult to accept that there is nothing that can bring the loved one back. During this stage, you might question God or make deals with yourself. It is common to find yourself going over things that occurred asking yourself "what if".

DEPRESSION

Grief can evoke strong emotions like pain and disease. Over time, grief comes in waves and the pain can be extreme. If you ever feel like life no longer holds any meaning, contact 911 immediately for help.

ACCEPTANCE

Grief can make you feel like nothing will ever be "right" again. It is important to know that as time passes, the pain eases. You will learn how to live again while keeping memories of those who have passed.

" HABAKKUK

1 I will stand upon my watch, and set me upon the tower, and will watch to see what he will say unto me, and what I shall answer when I am reproved.

2 And the LORD answered me, and said, Write the vision, and make it plain upon tables, that he may run that readeth it.

3 For the vision is yet for an appointed time, but at the end it shall speak, and not lie: though it tarry, wait for it; because it will surely come, it will not tarry.

4 Behold, his soul which is lifted up is not upright in him: but the just shall live by his faith.

make it plain

My Stages of Grief & Loss

Reflect on what you have learned about the five stages of grief and loss. Often, these stages happen in that exact order listed on *The Five Stages of Grief* page and they are typically experienced in waves. These waves can make a person feel like nothing will ever be the "right" again. However, people find that pain eases and it is possible to accept what has happen and move forward with life. Briefly describe what these situations looked like for you at each stage. Remember, if you have not experienced a specific stage listed below that is fine. If it's difficult for you to complete this worksheet, remember that grief and loss happens in many forms such as losing a person or losing a job and know that grief and loss is a process and it takes time. You will get there.

Denial: "I can't belive this is happening?"

Anger: "Why is this happening?"

Bargaining: "I will do anything to change what's happening?"

Depression: "I don't want to go on, what is the point?"

Acceptance: "I recognized what has happened and I realize that I cannot change it. Now it is time to work through this and cope".

THE PROCESS OF MOURNING

After a loved one is lost, it is difficult to face the pain of grief and a new world without their loved one. Mourning is the process of adapting to the changes that come with loss through a four-step process listed below.

ACCEPT THE REALITY OF THE LOSS

After a death, it's common to deny the situation or minimize the loss. To move forward from this step, the reality of the loss must be accepted.

PROCESS THE PAIN OF GRIEF

Grief involves hurtful emotions like sadness, anger, and guilt. It can be easier to avoid your feelings or bury them. However, it is best to confront your feelings and face them directly.

ADJUST TO YOUR NEW NORMAL

The death of a loved one can bring about many life adjustments such as internal adjustments like "Who am I now?", external adjustments like taking on new roles at work or spiritual adjustments that challenge your beliefs, values, and assumptions.

REMEMBER THE DECEASED

To move forward with your life doesn't mean you're forgetting the deceased. Finding a space in your thoughts that still leaves space for others is best. Completing this step means finding a healthy harmony between cherishing their memory and moving forward.

Session Reflection

During this session, you learned about the thoughts, feelings, and behaviors connected to the loss of something or someone important. You learned about the grieving process, the five stages of grief and loss, as well as how to identify how you are currently navigating or will navigate your mourning process. Below, ask yourself these questions and use the designated area to share your thoughts.

- Have I given myself permission to grieve at my own pace in the ways I needed to?
- Have I allowed myself to experience happiness without guilt since the loss of something or someone important?
- Have I expressed my honest feelings with others about the loss?
- Which stage of grief has been the most challenging for me and why?
- Have I considered seeking the help of a licensed therapist to support me during this grieving process?

05 HEALTHY RELATIONSHIPS

Healthy Relationships are an important part of a healthy balanced life. Every relationship has it's own norms and rituals. In any relationship, it's important to consider the foundation of your relationship. Are you able to communicate without being disrupted? Can you share your darkest secrets within the relationship without fear of them being exposed? Do you feel that you are loved? Is the person kind to you?

If you're ever unclear about how you should be treated in a relationship, think about your relationship with God. God is a provider, protector, and will always make sure your needs are met. How does your relationships align with how God sees you?

Remember, God did not create you to live in isolation without social connection. Research has shown that social interactions are critical for both mental and physical wellbeing. In fact, healthy relationships empower us to have better health outcomes, engage in healthy behaviors, and decrease the risk of heart-related illnesses and stress-related diseases.

you are worthy

Healthy Relationships

What are the components of a healthy relationship?

Did you know that healthy relationships take effort and compromise from both people? In fact, both parties should feel equally important and heard within the relationship dynamic. Another important factor in a relationship is the ability to be independent without fear of retaliation from the other person. Remember, its a good thing to have your own identify outside a relationship, as well as the confidence to make your own decisions within the relationship.

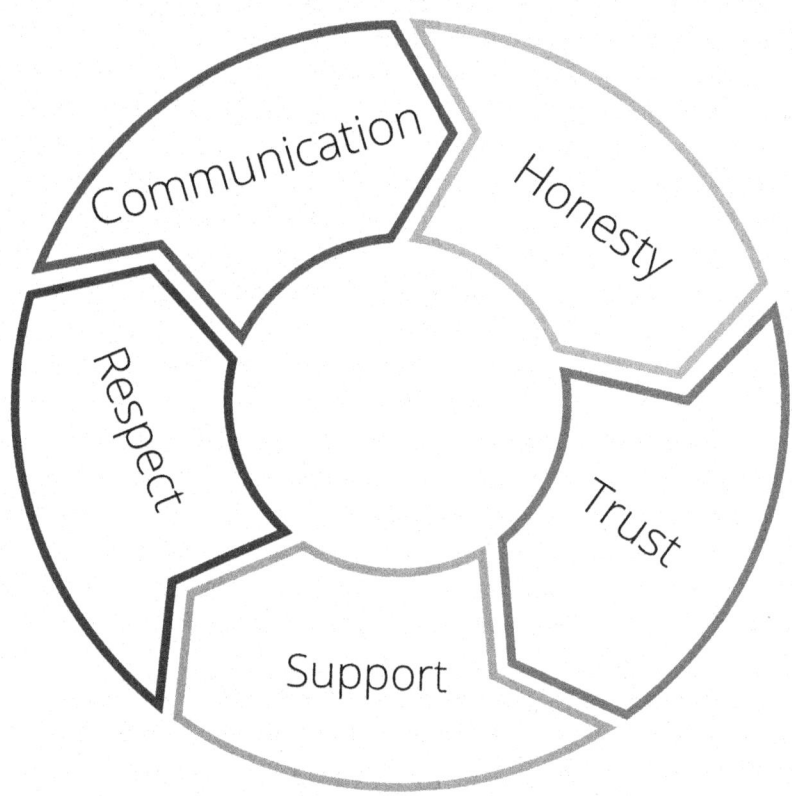

Think about what makes you happy and fulfilled outside of your relationships. What activities do you enjoy? What brings you peace? Think about incorporating a daily routine that involves activities that help you be the best version of yourself. Such as listening to inspirational podcasts, yoga, exercise, journaling or getting enough rest. What would your ideal daily routine look like?

WWW.FAITHSOARSCOUNSELING.COM

> **1 CORINTHIANS 13**

4 Love is patient and kind; love does not envy or boast; it is not arrogant or rude.

5 It does not insist on its own way; it is not irritable or resentful;

6 it does not rejoice at wrongdoing, but rejoices with the truth.

7 Love bears all things, believes all things, hopes all things, endures all things.

love is kind

Healthy Relationships

Are your relationships healthy?

You've learned that healthy relationships involve honesty, trust, respect, support, and communication. Now, it's time to evaluate your current relationships. In this activity, you will reflect on what works and what does not work in your current relationships. Keep in mind that you will have relationships that push you and pull you. For example, the relationship you may have with your mentee will involve you coaching them, offering your support, and helping them develop new skills (pulling them). On the other hand, the relationship you have with your mentor will involve them encouraging you to step outside your comfort zone and gain confidence in a new area (pushing you).

My desired Goal or Outcome in my relationships:

Help others without sacrificing my own well-being

To achieve this, I will need to:

Stop Doing	Prioritizing the needs of others before my own. It is important that I have energy to do the things that make me happy and fulfilled. I cant pour from an empty cup.
Do Less	Giving more than I can afford to mentally, physically, and emotionally. I want to make it a priority to listen to my body and understand what I am capable of not giving.
Keep Doing	Empower others through encouragement, positive affirmations, and active listening. I can do this by sharing inspirational podcasts, youtube videos, or books with my loved ones.
Start Doing	Develop strong boundaries to protect my emotional, mental and physically well-being. I do not want to say yes to helping someone when it means that I am saying no to myself.
Do More	Do more with less effort. Instead of going into debt helping my friend pay bills, I could help my friend secure a steady job by helping them create a LinkedIn profile and updated resume.

WWW.FAITHSOARSCOUNSELING.COM

Healthy Relationships

Your Turn

Think about a relationship that is not working for you. Identify a desired goal or outcome for the relationship. Next, share how you will achieve this goal. What will you stop doing? What will you do less? What will you keep doing? What will you start doing? What will you do more of?

My desired Goal or Outcome in my relationships:

To achieve this, I will need to:

Stop Doing	
Do Less	
Keep Doing	
Start Doing	
Do More	

WWW.FAITHSOARSCOUNSELING.COM

Types of Relationships
Are your relationships healthy?

There are five basic types of relationships: family, acquaintanceships, platonic, romantic and professional. Keep in mind that relationships constantly evolve and some relationships might overlap or coincide with one another. As you learn more about healthy relationships, think about the role each type of relationship plays in your life. Do you feel loved and supported by your family relationships? Are you fulfilled by your professional relationships? Have you made any promising romantic connections? What about your platonic relationships, are they reciprocal, loving or kind?

Family — 01
A group of individuals living together, typically united through ancestry or a particular bond. A family relationship can be categorized as nuclear family, single parent family, extended family, step family or grandparent family.

Acquaintance — 02
A relationship that is less intimate than a friend. Typically, this relationship is formed through school, work, church or common interest.

Platonic — 03
A supportive relationship in which people share a close bond but do not have a sexual relationship. Specific characteristics of a healthy friendship consists of trustworthiness, kindness, consideration, non-judgmental, uplifting, honesty and a good listener.

Romantic — 04
A voluntary relationship that is monogamous between individuals who have developed a unique bond based on emotional connection. Typically, these relationships are classified as boyfriend/girlfriend/significant other or simply "partner".

Professional — 05
A relationship that is solely for the purpose of meeting the expectations of your job. A good work relationship requires trust, respect, inclusion, communication and accountability. These relationships can be categorized as transactional or transformational.

Healthy Relationships

	What does a unhealthy and healthy relationship look like in your daily life? and Why do you consider it unhealthy or healthy?	Is this relationship an imbalance of power? Can you make your own decisions without fear of retaliation from the person?
Example	I consider the relationship I have with my grandmother healthy. I can trust her and she empowers me on the regular basis. I consider the relationship with my boyfriend unhealthy because he calls me out of my name and throws things at me when he is upset.	No, the relationship with my grandmother is not an imbalance of power. It is rooted in trust, respect, honestly and open communication. She truly loves me and wants the best for me. I hate to say this, but there is an imbalance of power between my boyfriend and I. He says he loves me, but it is hard to tell because his actions are different from his words. This causes my emotions to go up and down which makes me feel emotionally numb and tired.
Family		
Acquaintance		
Platonic		
Romantic		
Professional		

Yearly Vision

Take some quiet time to reflect on what you'd like to work during the next 12 months. Describe what your ideal life would look like and write down your initial thoughts on the steps you will need to take to get there. What are the key relationships you need to be successful? Is it a mentor? or Is it someone positive in your life? If you run-out of space, use notebook paper. This worksheet is designed to give you an idea of what you want. You may think that you don't need to write it down, but writing your goals down makes it more real and creates a commitment that compels you to move forward to achieve your goals. Try it!

Career	Finance
Relationships	**Love**
Personal Growth	**Health**
Recreation	**Spirituality**

Session Reflection

During this session, you learned about healthy relationships which are formed on honestly, trust, respect, support, and communication. You learned how to identify the healthy relationships in your life and the relationships that aren't so healthy. Below, ask yourself these questions and use the designated area to share your thoughts.

- What are my best traits in a healthy relationship with my family, friends and partner?
- What are some of the challenges of being in a relationship with me? This includes my platonic relationships and romantic relationships.
- Do I place more importance on my needs and wants within my relationships?
- What traumas am I carrying around from my previous relationships? Have I created an emotional space for someone new to enter my life?

Love Notes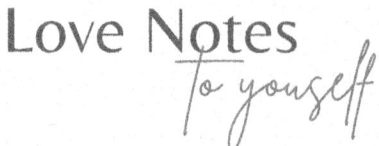
to yourself

Sis, you've grown so much since you started this self-healing journey. You've learned techniques for managing stress more effectively to enjoy your life as well as how to manage anxiety to live fearlessly! You've learned how to overcome loss and move forward. Most of all, you've learned how to overcome limiting beliefs and how to break the cycle of unhealthy relationships. Now, it's time to soar and embrace the new you. Below, write a love note to yourself. How do you think you've grown? Which lesson has helped you the most? What are you most proud of? Remember, you got this and I will be here for you!

_____
_____
_____
_____
_____
_____
_____
_____
_____
_____
_____
_____
_____
_____
_____
_____
_____
_____
_____
_____
_____
_____
_____
_____
_____

worksheets *extra*

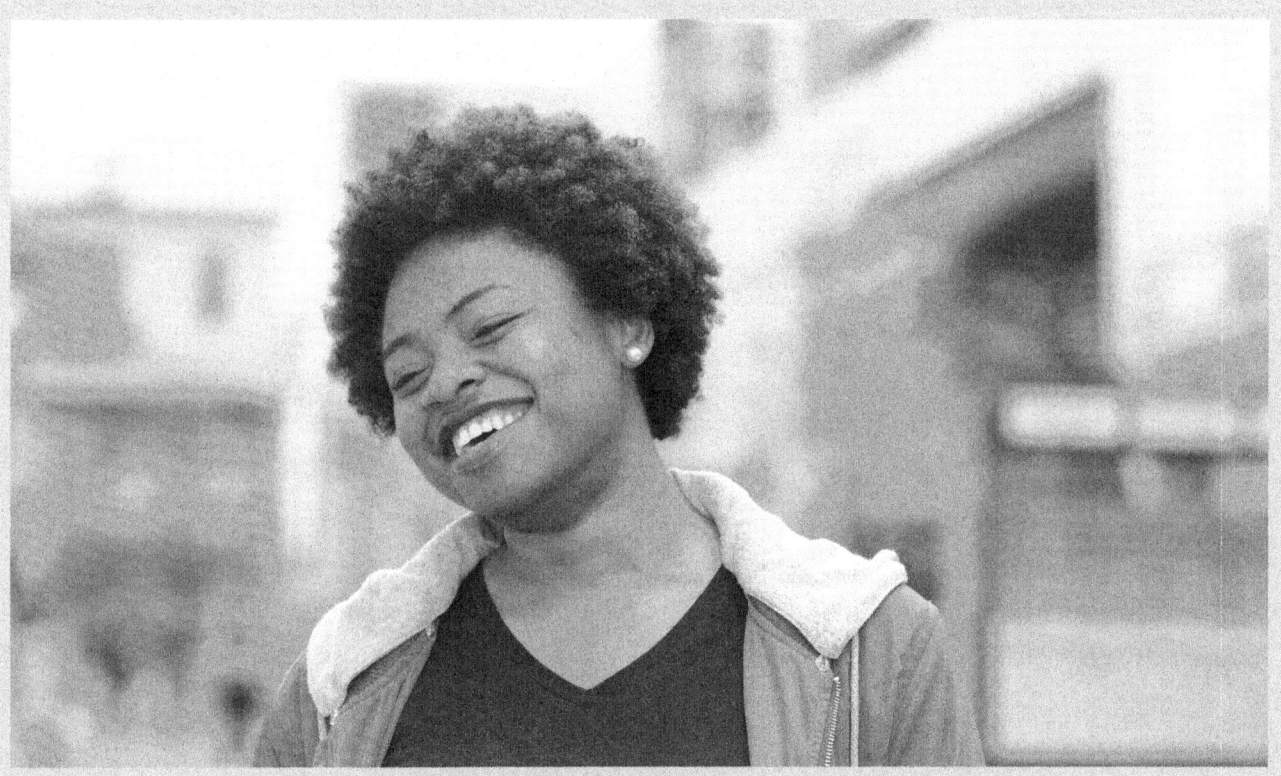

"Be strong and of a good courage, fear not, nor be afraid of them: for the Lord thy God, he it is that doth go with thee; he will not fail thee, nor forsake thee".

Deuteronomy 31:6 (KJV)

Weekly Success Planner

Weekly planning will keep you motivated, help you perform at a higher level, measuring your progress, and most of all it will help you prioritize. Use this blank template to identify a long-term goal, your weekly priorities and why they're important to you. Once you have completed the activity, consider purchasing a yearly calendar to help you practice effective time management. Sis, let's plan for success!

Long Term Goal/s: usually take 12 months or more to achieve

make your weekly priorities align with this goal:

My Weekly Priorities:

01.

02.

03.

Why they're Important to me:

Potential Distractions

How to Avoid Them

Other Notes

Weekly Success Planner

Weekly planning will keep you motivated, help you perform at a higher level, measuring your progress, and most of all it will help you prioritize. Use this blank template to identify a long-term goal, your weekly priorities and why they're important to you. Once you have completed the activity, consider purchasing a yearly calendar to help you practice effective time management. Sis, let's plan for success!

Long Term Goal/s: usually take 12 months or more to achieve

make your weekly priorities align with this goal:

My Weekly Priorities:

01

02

03

Why they're Important to me:

Potential Distractions

How to Avoid Them

Other Notes

Healthy Relationships

Your Turn

Think about a relationship that is not working for you. Identify a desired goal or outcome for the relationship. Next, share how you will achieve this goal. What will you stop doing? What will you do less? What will you keep doing? What will you start doing? What will you do more of?

My desired Goal or Outcome in my relationships:

To achieve this, I will need to:

Stop Doing

Do Less

Keep Doing

Start Doing

Do More

WWW.FAITHSOARSCOUNSELING.COM

Healthy Relationships

Your Turn

Think about a relationship that is not working for you. Identify a desired goal or outcome for the relationship. Next, share how you will achieve this goal. What will you stop doing? What will you do less? What will you keep doing? What will you start doing? What will you do more of?

My desired Goal or Outcome in my relationships:

To achieve this, I will need to:

Stop Doing

Do Less

Keep Doing

Start Doing

Do More

WWW.FAITHSOARSCOUNSELING.COM

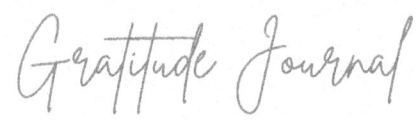

Morning:

I am greatful for:

I'm looking forward to:

Daily Affirmations:

Evening:

Good things that happened today:

Things I can do to make tomorrow even better:

Gratitude Journal

Morning:

I am greatful for:

I'm looking forward to:

Daily Affirmations:

Evening:

Good things that happened today:

Things I can do to make tomorrow even better:

Session Reflection

Session Reflection

Love Notes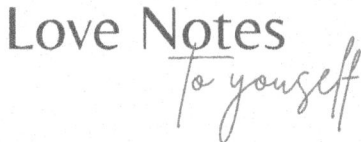

Sis, you've grown so much since you started this self-healing journey. You've learned techniques for managing stress more effectively to enjoy your life as well as how to manage anxiety to live fearlessly! You've learned how to overcome loss and move forward. Most of all, you've learned how to overcome limiting beliefs and how to break the cycle of unhealthy relationships. Now, it's time to soar and embrace the new you. Below, write a love note to yourself. How do you think you've grown? Which lesson has helped you the most? What are you most proud of? Remember, you got this and I will be here for you!

_____
_____
_____
_____
_____
_____
_____
_____
_____
_____
_____
_____
_____
_____
_____
_____
_____
_____
_____
_____
_____
_____
_____
_____
_____
_____

Love Notes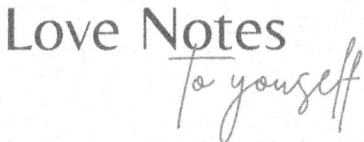
to yourself

Sis, you've grown so much since you started this self-healing journey. You've learned techniques for managing stress more effectively to enjoy your life as well as how to manage anxiety to live fearlessly! You've learned how to overcome loss and move forward. Most of all, you've learned how to overcome limiting beliefs and how to break the cycle of unhealthy relationships. Now, it's time to soar and embrace the new you. Below, write a love note to yourself. How do you think you've grown? Which lesson has helped you the most? What are you most proud of? Remember, you got this and I will be here for you!

_____
_____
_____
_____
_____
_____
_____
_____
_____
_____
_____
_____
_____
_____
_____
_____
_____
_____
_____
_____
_____
_____
_____
_____

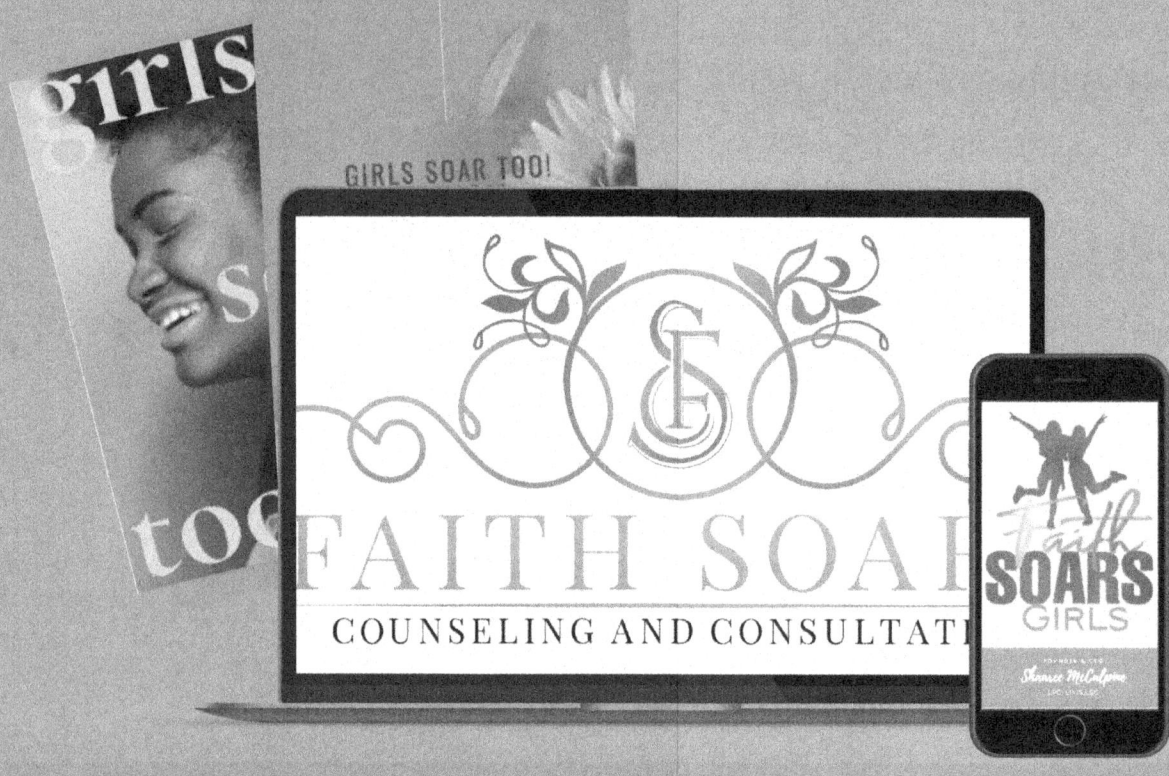

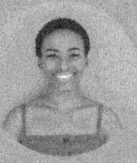 

I had no one to turn to (*outside of God*) until I met Shaaree McCalpine. I learned so much and most importantly learned how to take care of me. I had to learn that it is ok to not always be the go-to person and that my NO was a full sentence."

BOOK WITH FAITH SOARS

Faith Soars Counseling Services is a Christian based counseling practice that will help you learn to cope with stressful situations, goal setting, anxiety, depression, self-esteem and how to cope with grief and loss.

SCHEDULE APPOINTMENT

References

Stress

1. DeLongis, A., Coyne, J. C., Dakof, G., Folkman, S., & Lazarus, R. S. (1982). Relationship of daily hassles, uplifts, and major life events to health status. Health psychology, 1(2), 119.

2. Larsson, U. G., Ohlsson, A., Berglund, A. K., & Nilsson, S. (2017). Daily uplifts and coping as a buffer against everyday hassles: Relationship with stress reactions over time in military personnel.

3. Lu, L. (1991). Daily hassles and mental health: A longitudinal study. British Journal of Psychology, 82(4), 441-447.

4. Pinquart, M., & Sörensen, S. (2003). Associations of stressors and uplifts of caregiving with caregiver burden and depressive mood: a meta-analysis. The Journals of Gerontology Series B: Psychological Sciences and Social Sciences, 58(2), 112-128.

5. Totenhagen, C. J., Serido, J., Curran, M. A., & Butler, E. A. (2012). Daily hassles and uplifts: A diary study on understanding relationship quality. Journal of Family Psychology, 26(5), 719.

6. Windle, G. (2011). What is resilience? A review and concept analysis. Reviews in Clinical Gerontology, 21(2), 152-169.

References

Anxiety

1. DeLongis, A., Coyne, J. C., Dakof, G., Folkman, S., & Lazarus, R. S. (1982). Relationship of daily hassles, uplifts, and major life events to health status. Health psychology, 1(2), 119.

2. Larsson, U. G., Ohlsson, A., Berglund, A. K., & Nilsson, S. (2017). Daily uplifts and coping as a buffer against everyday hassles: Relationship with stress reactions over time in military personnel.

3. Lu, L. (1991). Daily hassles and mental health: A longitudinal study. British Journal of Psychology, 82(4), 441-447.

4. Pinquart, M., & Sörensen, S. (2003). Associations of stressors and uplifts of caregiving with caregiver burden and depressive mood: a meta-analysis. The Journals of Gerontology Series B: Psychological Sciences and Social Sciences, 58(2), 112-128.

5. Totenhagen, C. J., Serido, J., Curran, M. A., & Butler, E. A. (2012). Daily hassles and uplifts: A diary study on understanding relationship quality. Journal of Family Psychology, 26(5), 719.

6. Windle, G. (2011). What is resilience? A review and concept analysis. Reviews in Clinical Gerontology, 21(2), 152-169.

References

Depression

1. American Psychiatric Association. (2013). Diagnostic and statistical manual of mental disorders (DSM-5®). American Psychiatric Pub.

2. Andrade, L., Caraveo-Anduaga, J. J., Berglund, P., Bijl, R. V., Graaf, R. D., Vollebergh, W., ... & Kawakami, N. (2003). The epidemiology of major depressive episodes: results from the International Consortium of Psychiatric Epidemiology (ICPE) Surveys. International journal of methods in psychiatric research, 12(1), 3-21.

3. Driessen, E., & Hollon, S. D. (2010). Cognitive behavioral therapy for mood disorders: efficacy, moderators and mediators. Psychiatric Clinics, 33(3), 537-555.

4. Hirschfeld, R. M. (2001). The comorbidity of major depression and anxiety disorders: recognition and management in primary care. Primary care companion to the Journal of clinical psychiatry, 3(6), 244.

5. Isometsä, E. (2014). Suicidal behaviour in mood disorders—who, when, and why?. The Canadian Journal of Psychiatry, 59(3), 120-130.

6. Kirsch, I., Deacon, B. J., Huedo-Medina, T. B., Scoboria, A., Moore, T. J., & Johnson, B. T. (2008). Initial severity and antidepressant benefits: a meta-analysis of data submitted to the Food and Drug Administration. PLoS medicine, 5(2), e45.

7. Paluska, S. A., & Schwenk, T. L. (2000). Physical activity and mental health. Sports medicine, 29(3), 167-180.

References

Grief & Loss

1. Kübler-Ross, E. (2009). On death and dying: What the dying have to teach doctors, nurses, clergy and their own families. Taylor & Francis.

2. Bruce, C. A. (2007). Helping patients, families, caregivers, and physicians, in the grieving process. The Journal of the American Osteopathic Association, 107(Suppl. 7), ES33-ES40.

3. Worden, J. W. (2018). Grief counseling and grief therapy, fifth edition: A handbook for the mental health practitioner. Springer Publishing Company.

4. American Psychiatric Association. (2013). Diagnostic and statistical manual of mental disorders (5th ed.).

5. Neimeyer, R.A. (2000). Searching for the meaning of meaning: Grief therapy and the process of reconstruction. Death Studies, 24, 541-558.

6. Versalle, A., & McDowell, E. E. (2005). The attitudes of men and women concerning gender differences in grief. OMEGA-Journal of Death and Dying, 50(1), 53-67.

7. Zisook, S., & Shear, K. (2009). Grief and bereavement: what psychiatrists need to know. World Psychiatry, 8(2), 67-74.

References

Healthy Relationships

1. P. Greeff, Tanya De Bruyne, A. (2000). Conflict management style and marital satisfaction. Journal of Sex & Marital Therapy, 26(4), 321-334.

2. Bruce, C. A. (2007). Helping patients, families, caregivers, and physicians, in the grieving process. The Journal of the American Osteopathic Association, 107(Suppl. 7), ES33-ES40.

3. Gordon, C. L., Arnette, R. A., & Smith, R. E. (2011). Have you thanked your spouse today?: Felt and expressed gratitude among married couples. Personality and Individual Differences, 50(3), 339-343.

4. Woody Schuldt, LMHC. "The Benefits of MINDFULNESS (ARTICLE)." Therapist Aid, Therapist Aid, 29 Apr. 2016, www.therapistaid.com/therapy-article/benefits-of-mindfulness.

5. 'Healthy Relationships'.Https://Www.therapistaid.com/Therapy-Worksheet/Boundaries-Discussion-Questions.

6. "Healthy Relationships." The Hotline, 22 Oct. 2020, www.thehotline.org/resources/healthy-relationships/.

COPYRIGHT NOTICE

All rights reserved. No part of this workbook may be reproduced or used in any manner without the prior written permission of the copyright owner, Shaaree M. McCalpine except for the use of brief quotations in a workbook review.

Shaaree xoxo

COUNSELOR | COACH | CEO